Comprehensive Guide to Weight Loss

Chapter 1: Introduction to Weight Loss

Weight loss is the process of losing body weight by reducing the amount of fat stored in the body. It can be achieved through a combination of diet and exercise, as well as other lifestyle changes. Losing weight can have numerous health benefits, including reduced risk of obesity-related conditions such as heart disease, diabetes, and some cancers. It can also improve self-esteem, boost energy levels, and enhance physical performance.

The role of diet and exercise in weight loss cannot be overstated. A healthy diet that is low in calories and high in nutrients can help to reduce body fat, while regular physical activity can help to burn calories and increase muscle mass. Together, diet and exercise can help to boost metabolism and increase the rate at which the body burns calories.

However, it's important to remember that weight loss is not a quick or easy process. It requires consistent effort and patience, as well as a willingness to make sustainable lifestyle changes. Crash diets or fad workouts may promise rapid results, but they are often not sustainable or healthy in the long run. Instead, it is important to adopt a balanced and realistic approach to weight loss that focuses on making healthy lifestyle choices.

One key to successful weight loss is setting realistic goals. This means determining a healthy weight range for your age, gender, and height, and setting achievable goals for losing weight at a safe and sustainable pace. Losing 1-2 pounds per week is generally considered a healthy rate of weight loss, although this may vary depending on individual factors.

In addition to setting realistic goals, it is also important to understand the role of nutrition in weight loss. This means learning about the different types of macronutrients (carbohydrates, proteins, and fats) and micronutrients (vitamins and minerals) that the body needs to function properly, as well as how to choose healthy sources of these nutrients. Reading food labels and understanding serving sizes can also help to ensure that you are making informed choices about what you eat.

Meal planning and prep can also play a crucial role in weight loss success. Planning ahead and cooking at home can help to ensure that you have healthy, low-calorie options available, and can help to prevent impulsive or unhealthy food choices. Simple, healthy recipes that are easy to prepare can make meal planning and prep more manageable.

Incorporating exercise into your weight loss journey is also essential. Regular physical activity can help to burn calories, increase muscle mass, and boost metabolism. There are many different types of exercise to choose from, including cardio, strength training, and high-intensity interval training (HIIT). It is important to find activities that you enjoy and that fit your lifestyle, and to create a balanced exercise routine that includes a variety of different activities.

Finally, it is important to be prepared for common challenges that may arise during your weight loss journey. Dealing with cravings and emotional eating, staying motivated and accountable, and managing stress and getting enough sleep can all be challenges. But by learning how to overcome these challenges and adopting healthy habits, you can stay on track and achieve your weight loss goals.

In this book, we will delve deeper into each of these topics and provide specific, actionable tips and strategies for successful weight loss. We will also discuss the importance of maintenance and lifelong habits, and provide guidance on how to maintain your weight loss and adopt healthy habits for the long term. By the end of this book, you will have the tools and knowledge you need to successfully lose weight and improve your overall health.

Chapter 2: Setting Realistic Goals

One key to successful weight loss is setting realistic goals. This means determining a healthy weight range for your age, gender, and height, and setting achievable goals for losing weight at a safe and sustainable pace.

To determine a healthy weight range, you can use a body mass index (BMI) calculator or consult with a healthcare professional. BMI is a measure of body fat based on height and weight, and is used to classify people into categories such as underweight, normal weight, overweight, and obese. However, it's important to note that BMI is not always a reliable indicator of health, as it does not take into account factors such as muscle mass, bone density, and distribution of fat. Therefore, it's a good idea to discuss your weight goals with a healthcare professional, who can take into account your individual circumstances and provide personalized guidance. They can also help to assess your overall health and identify any potential risks or concerns that may need to be addressed as part of your weight loss journey.

Once you have determined a healthy weight range, you can set achievable goals for losing weight. Losing 1-2 pounds per week is generally considered a healthy rate of weight loss, although this may vary depending on individual factors such as starting weight, age, and activity level. It's important to be patient and consistent, and to focus on making sustainable lifestyle changes rather than seeking quick fixes. Crash diets or fad workouts may promise rapid results, but they are often not sustainable or healthy in the long run. Instead, aim to make gradual, sustainable changes that you can maintain over time. Remember that losing weight is a journey, not a destination, and it's important to focus on the process rather than just the end result.

In addition to setting specific weight loss goals, it's also helpful to set smaller, achievable goals along the way. For example, you might set a goal to exercise for 30 minutes every day, or to try a new healthy recipe once a week. These smaller goals can help to keep you motivated and on track, and can help you see progress even if you are not losing weight as quickly as you had hoped. Celebrating your progress and accomplishments, no matter how small, can help to keep you motivated and encourage you to continue making healthy choices.

It's also important to be realistic about the time and effort it will take to reach your weight loss goals. Losing weight requires a commitment to healthy habits and lifestyle changes, and it's important to be prepared for the challenges that may arise along the way. Dealing with cravings and emotional eating, staying motivated and accountable, and managing stress and getting enough sleep can all be challenges. But by learning how to overcome these challenges and adopting healthy habits, you can stay on track and achieve your weight loss goals.

Staying motivated and accountable can be particularly important when it comes to weight loss. Seeking support from friends, family, or a healthcare professional can help to keep you on track, and can provide a sense of accountability and encouragement. You might also consider joining a weight loss group or seeking the guidance of a registered dietitian or personal trainer. These professionals can provide expert advice and support, and can help you develop a personalized weight loss plan that is tailored to your needs and goals.

Another way to stay motivated and accountable is to track your progress. This can be as simple as keeping a food diary or journal to record your meals and activities, or using a tracking app or device to monitor your calorie intake, exercise, and other habits. Seeing your progress in writing or numbers can be a powerful motivator, and can help you stay on track.

Chapter 3: Understanding Nutrition

Understanding nutrition is an essential part of any weight loss journey. The types of foods and beverages you consume can have a major impact on your weight and overall health, and making informed choices about what you eat can help you achieve your weight loss goals and maintain a healthy weight.

There are three main types of macronutrients (nutrients that provide energy) that the body needs to function properly: carbohydrates, proteins, and fats. These nutrients provide the body with energy, and they also play important roles in supporting various bodily functions and processes.

Carbohydrates are the body's primary source of energy, and they are found in a wide variety of foods, including grains, fruits, vegetables, dairy products, and legumes. There are two main types of carbohydrates: simple carbs and complex carbs. Simple carbs are found in sugary foods and beverages, and they are quickly absorbed by the body. Complex carbs are found in whole grains, vegetables, and other high-fiber foods, and they are absorbed more slowly, providing a sustained source of energy.

Proteins are important for building and repairing tissues, and they are also necessary for the production of hormones, enzymes, and other substances in the body. Proteins can be found in animal sources such as meat, poultry, fish, and dairy products, as well as in plant sources such as legumes, nuts, and seeds. It's important to include a variety of protein sources in your diet to ensure that you are getting all of the necessary amino acids (the building blocks of protein).

Fats are a type of macronutrient that provides energy and helps to support cell growth and development. Fats are also necessary for the absorption of certain vitamins and minerals. There are several types of fats, including saturated fats, unsaturated fats, and trans fats. Saturated fats are found in animal products such as meat and dairy, and they are solid at room temperature. Unsaturated fats are found in plant-based sources such as nuts, seeds, and vegetable oils, and they are liquid at room temperature. Trans fats are found in processed and fried foods, and they have been linked to a range of health problems. It's important to choose healthy sources of fats, and to limit your intake of saturated and trans fats.

In addition to macronutrients, the body also needs micronutrients (vitamins and minerals) to function properly. These nutrients are necessary for a wide range of bodily processes, and they are found in a variety of foods. Some key micronutrients to focus on include:

Vitamins:

- There are several types of vitamins, including fat-soluble vitamins (such as A, D, E, and K).
- Vitamin A: This vitamin is important for vision, immune function, and skin health. It can be found in animal sources such as liver, eggs, and dairy products, as well as in plant sources such as sweet potatoes, carrots, and dark leafy greens.
- Vitamin D: This vitamin is important for bone health and immune function, and it can be synthesized by the body when the skin is exposed to sunlight. It can also be found in animal sources such as fatty fish, egg yolks, and fortified foods such as milk and cereal.

- Vitamin E: This vitamin is an antioxidant that helps to protect cells from damage, and it can be found in plant-based oils, nuts, seeds, and leafy greens.
- Vitamin K: This vitamin is important for blood clotting and bone health, and it can be found in leafy greens, broccoli, and other vegetables.
- Minerals: There are several minerals that are important for good health, including calcium, iron, sodium, and potassium.
- Calcium: This mineral is important for bone health, and it can be found in dairy products, leafy greens, and fortified foods such as orange juice and tofu.
- Iron: This mineral is important for carrying oxygen in the blood, and it can be found in animal sources such as red meat, poultry, and seafood, as well as in plant sources such as beans, nuts, and leafy greens.
- Sodium: This mineral is important for maintaining fluid balance in the body, and it is found in many processed and packaged foods. It's important to consume sodium in moderation, as high levels can contribute to high blood pressure and other health problems.
- Potassium: This mineral is important for maintaining proper heart function and regulating blood pressure, and it can be found in fruits, vegetables, and dairy products.

It's important to consume a balanced diet that includes a variety of different nutrients to ensure that your body is getting all of the nourishment it needs. This means choosing a variety of different types of foods, including whole grains, fruits and vegetables, lean proteins, and healthy fats. Reading food labels and understanding serving sizes can also help to ensure that you are making informed choices about what you eat.

In addition to understanding the types of nutrients your body needs, it's also important to be mindful of portion sizes. Consuming too many calories, regardless of the source, can contribute to weight gain. On the other hand, consuming too few calories can lead to nutrient deficiencies and other health problems. A registered dietitian or healthcare professional can help you determine an appropriate calorie intake for your individual needs and goals.

By understanding nutrition and making informed choices about what you eat, you can support your weight loss goals and maintain a healthy weight. Remember to focus on consuming a balanced diet that includes a variety of different nutrients, and to be mindful of portion sizes. With the right nutrition and lifestyle habits, you can achieve your weight loss goals and enjoy.

Chapter 4: Meal Planning and Prep

Incorporating physical activity into your weight loss journey can help you burn calories, build muscle, and improve your overall health. Regular exercise can also help to boost your mood, reduce stress, and improve sleep quality.

There are many different types of physical activity to choose from, and the best type of exercise for you will depend on your individual preferences and goals. Some options include:

Cardio: Cardio exercises, also known as aerobic exercises, involve sustained, rhythmic movements that increase your heart rate and improve cardiovascular endurance. Examples of cardio exercises include running, cycling, swimming, and dancing. Cardio exercises are a great way to burn calories and improve your overall fitness, and they can be done at a variety of intensity levels to suit your fitness level and goals.

Strength training: Strength training exercises involve using resistance to build muscle mass and strength. Examples of strength training exercises include weight lifting, bodyweight exercises (such as push-ups and squats), and resistance band exercises. Strength training is important for maintaining muscle mass and strength, which can help to boost metabolism and support weight loss. It's a good idea to include strength training exercises at least two days per week, as part of a well-rounded fitness routine.

Flexibility: Flexibility exercises, also known as stretching exercises, involve stretching and lengthening the muscles to improve range of motion and reduce the risk of injury. Examples of flexibility exercises include yoga, tai chi, and Pilates. Incorporating flexibility exercises into your routine can help to improve your overall range of motion and reduce muscle stiffness, and they can be particularly beneficial for people who sit for long periods of time.

Balance and coordination: Balance and coordination exercises involve using different parts of the body together to improve balance, coordination, and body awareness. Examples of balance and coordination exercises include tai chi, yoga, and certain types of dance. These types of exercises can be especially helpful for older adults, who may be at risk of falls, and they can also be beneficial for improving athletic performance.

It's important to find physical activities that you enjoy, as this will make it more likely that you will stick with them in the long run. It's also a good idea to mix up your workouts and try different types of exercises to keep things interesting and to challenge your body in different ways. This can help to prevent boredom and plateaus, and can also help to improve overall fitness and performance.

The Centers for Disease Control and Prevention (CDC) recommends adults aim for at least 150 minutes of moderate-intensity aerobic exercise or 75 minutes of vigorous-intensity aerobic exercise per week, along with strength training exercises at least two days per week. This can be broken up into shorter sessions of 10-15 minutes throughout the week, or longer sessions of 30-60 minutes. It's important to listen to your body and not push yourself too hard, especially when starting a new exercise routine. Consult with a healthcare professional or a certified personal trainer if you have any concerns or injuries.

Incorporating physical activity into your weight loss journey can have numerous benefits, and it's an important part of maintaining a healthy weight and overall health. By finding activities that you enjoy and mixing up your workouts, you can make exercise a sustainable and enjoyable part of your routine. It's also important to focus on making physical activity a part of your daily routine, rather than just an occasional event. This can help to make it a habit, and can help to ensure that you are getting regular exercise on a consistent basis.

In addition to traditional forms of exercise, there are also many other ways to incorporate physical activity into your daily routine. Some options include taking the stairs instead of the elevator, walking or cycling to work or errands, gardening, or even just going for a walk or hike in your free time. Every little bit of movement can add up and contribute to your overall fitness and health.

It's also important to consider the intensity of your workouts. High-intensity interval training (HIIT) involves short bursts of intense exercise followed by periods of rest, and it can be an effective way to boost fitness and burn calories. However, it's important to listen to your body and not push yourself too hard, especially if you are new to exercise. It's also a good idea to incorporate a warm-up and cool-down into your workouts to help prevent injury and improve overall performance.

Incorporating physical activity into your weight loss journey can be challenging, but it's an essential part of achieving and maintaining a healthy weight. By finding activities that you enjoy and making them a regular part of your routine, you can make exercise a sustainable and enjoyable part of your journey. Remember to listen to your body, and to consult with a healthcare professional or a certified personal trainer if you have any concerns or injuries. With the right mindset and approach, you can incorporate physical activity into your weight loss journey and enjoy all of the many benefits it has to offer.

Chapter 5: Incorporating Exercise

Losing weight and maintaining a healthy weight can be challenging, and it can be helpful to have a support system to help you along the way. A supportive network of friends, family, and healthcare professionals can provide encouragement, motivation, and guidance as you work towards your weight loss goals.

One way to build a support system is to seek out a weight loss group or program. Many communities offer support groups or structured weight loss programs that provide education, support, and accountability. These groups can be a great way to connect with others who are working towards similar goals, and they can provide a sense of community and belonging. Many weight loss groups also offer educational resources, such as nutrition and exercise guides, to help participants learn more about healthy habits and make informed choices about their diet and lifestyle.

Another way to build a support system is to enlist the help of friends and family. Having a supportive network of people who care about your well-being can be incredibly helpful, and they can provide encouragement and motivation as you work towards your goals. You may want to consider sharing your weight loss journey with a close friend or family member who can provide emotional support and accountability. You may also want to consider sharing your journey with your social media followers or by starting a blog or podcast. Sharing your journey with others can provide a sense of accountability and can also be a great way to connect with others who may be facing similar challenges.

It's also important to work with a healthcare professional as you work towards your weight loss goals. A registered dietitian or a healthcare provider can help you create a personalized weight loss plan that takes into account your individual needs and goals. They can provide guidance on nutrition and exercise, and can help you identify any potential barriers or challenges that may arise as you work towards your goals. They can also help you develop strategies for overcoming these challenges and staying on track.

In addition to seeking out external support, it's also important to focus on building self-awareness and self-compassion. This means being kind and understanding towards yourself as you work towards your goals, and recognizing that setbacks and challenges are a normal part of the process. It's important to be patient with yourself and to focus on the progress you have made, rather than dwelling on any setbacks or failures. It can be helpful to practice self-compassion by reminding yourself that everyone makes mistakes and that it's okay to ask for help when you need it.

Another way to build self-awareness and self-compassion is to practice mindfulness. Mindfulness is the practice of bringing your attention to the present moment, without judgment. It can be helpful to set aside time each day to practice mindfulness, whether through meditation, yoga, or simply by paying attention to your breath and your surroundings. Mindfulness can help to improve self-awareness and reduce stress, and it can be a helpful tool to have in your weight loss journey.

By building a supportive network of friends, family, and healthcare professionals, and by focusing on self-awareness and self-compassion, you can create a foundation of support as you work towards your weight loss goals. Remember to be kind and understanding towards yourself, and to focus on the progress you have made. With the right support system in place, you can feel more confident and motivated as you work towards your goals.

Here is some general guidance for different body types:

- Endomorph body type: Endomorphs tend to have a rounder, softer body type, and may have a harder time losing weight. An effective exercise plan for endomorphs may include a mix of cardio and strength training, with a focus on high-intensity interval training (HIIT) to boost metabolism. Endomorphs may also benefit from incorporating activities that involve sustained movement, such as swimming or cycling, to help burn calories.
- Ectomorph body type: Ectomorphs tend to have a slender, linear body type, and may have a harder time gaining weight. An effective exercise plan for ectomorphs may include a mix of strength training and hypertrophy (muscle-building) exercises, with a focus on increasing resistance over time. Ectomorphs may also benefit from incorporating rest days into their routine to allow their muscles time to recover and grow.
- Mesomorph body type: Mesomorphs tend to have a naturally athletic, muscular body type, and may find it easier to gain muscle and lose fat. An effective exercise plan for mesomorphs may include a mix of cardio, strength training, and flexibility exercises to help maintain overall fitness and health. Mesomorphs may also benefit from focusing on specific muscle groups or sports-specific training to improve performance in their chosen activity.

It's important to note that these are just general guidelines, and the best exercise plan for you will depend on your individual goals, preferences, and needs. It's also important to consult with a healthcare professional or a certified personal trainer before starting any new exercise program, especially if you have any underlying health conditions or injuries. They can help to create a personalized exercise plan that is tailored to your individual needs and goals.

In addition to following a structured exercise plan, it's also important to focus on overall lifestyle habits, such as getting enough sleep, managing stress, and consuming a balanced diet. These habits can have a significant impact on your overall health and fitness and can help to support your weight loss goals.

Remember to listen to your body and not push yourself too hard, and to consult with a healthcare professional or a certified personal trainer if you have any concerns or injuries. With the right exercise plan and lifestyle habits, you can achieve your weight loss goals and enjoy improved overall health and fitness.

Chapter 6: Overcoming Common Challenges

Losing weight and maintaining a healthy weight can be a challenging and often long-term process, and it's important to find ways to stay motivated along the way. Here are some tips for staying motivated on your weight loss journey:

- Set specific, achievable goals: Rather than setting a broad goal of "losing weight," try setting specific, achievable goals that you can work towards. For example, you might set a goal to lose 5% of your body weight within the next three months, or to increase your daily step count by 1,000 steps per day. Specific, achievable goals can provide a sense of direction and can help you stay motivated as you work towards them.
- Celebrate your progress: It's important to recognize and celebrate your progress as you work towards your weight loss goals. This could involve setting small rewards for yourself along the way, such as a new workout outfit or a massage. Celebrating your progress can help to keep you motivated and can also provide a sense of accomplishment as you work towards your goals.
- Find support: Having a support system of friends, family, and healthcare professionals can be incredibly helpful as you work towards your weight loss goals. A supportive network can provide encouragement, motivation, and guidance as you navigate the challenges of weight loss. Consider seeking out a weight loss group

or program, or sharing your journey with friends and family to create a foundation of support.

- Don't be too hard on yourself: It's important to be kind and understanding towards yourself as you work towards your weight loss goals. Setbacks and challenges are a normal part of the process, and it's important to be patient and to focus on the progress you have made, rather than dwelling on any setbacks or failures. It can be helpful to practice self-compassion and to remind yourself that everyone makes mistakes, and that it's okay to ask for help when you need it.
- Keep things interesting: It's important to mix up your workouts and try different types of exercises to keep things interesting and to challenge your body in different ways. This can help to prevent boredom and plateaus, and can also help to improve overall fitness and performance. Consider trying new activities or sports, joining a group fitness class, or trying out a new workout program or app to keep things fresh and exciting.
- Seek out inspiration: Sometimes, all it takes is a little bit of inspiration to keep us motivated. Consider seeking out motivation from sources such as inspiring quotes, motivational podcasts or books, or by following weight loss blogs or social media accounts. These sources can provide a boost of motivation when you need it most.
- By setting specific, achievable goals, celebrating your progress, seeking out support, being kind to yourself, and keeping things interesting, you can stay motivated on your weight loss journey. Remember to be patient and to focus on the progress you have made, and to seek out inspiration and motivation when you need it. With

the right mindset and approach, you can stay motivated and on track as you work towards your weight loss goals.

Chapter 7: Maintenance and Life Long Habits

Losing weight and maintaining a healthy weight can be a challenging and often long-term process, and it's normal to experience setbacks and challenges along the way. Here are some tips for navigating setbacks and challenges on your weight loss journey:

- Don't beat yourself up: It's important to be kind and understanding towards yourself as you work towards your weight loss goals. Setbacks and challenges are a normal part of the process, and it's important to be patient and to focus on the progress you have made, rather than dwelling on any setbacks or failures. It can be helpful to practice self-compassion and to remind yourself that everyone makes mistakes, and that it's okay to ask for help when you need it.
- Take a step back and reassess: If you are experiencing a setback or challenge, it can be helpful to take a step back and reassess your approach. Consider consulting with a healthcare professional or a certified personal trainer, or reviewing your diet and exercise plan to see if there are any adjustments that can be made. It's also a good idea to check in with yourself and see if there are any underlying emotional or psychological factors that may be contributing to your challenge.
- Find support: Having a support system of friends,

family, and healthcare professionals can be incredibly helpful as you work towards your weight loss goals. A supportive network can provide encouragement, motivation, and guidance as you navigate the challenges of weight loss. Consider seeking out a weight loss group or program, or sharing your journey with friends and family to create a foundation of support.

- Keep things in perspective: It's important to keep things in perspective as you work towards your weight loss goals. Remember that weight loss is a journey, and that setbacks and challenges are a normal part of the process. It's important to stay focused on your long-term goals and to keep working towards them, even when you experience setbacks or challenges.

By being kind to yourself, taking a step back and reassessing, seeking out support, and keeping things in perspective, you can navigate setbacks and challenges on your weight loss journey. Remember to be patient and to focus on the progress you have made, and to seek out help when you need it. With the right mindset and approach, you can overcome setbacks and challenges and stay on track towards your weight loss goals.

Losing weight and maintaining a healthy weight involves more than just a short-term diet or exercise program. It requires a commitment to making sustainable lifestyle changes that can support long-term weight loss and overall health. Here are some tips for maintaining your weight loss and building healthy habits for the long haul:

- Make sustainable changes: Rather than trying to make dramatic changes all at once, focus on making small, sustainable changes that you can stick to over the long term. This can help to build healthy habits that can support long-term weight loss and overall health. For example, rather than cutting out entire food groups or drastically reducing your calorie intake, try making small changes to your diet, such as choosing whole, unprocessed foods, reducing your intake of added sugars and saturated fats, and increasing your intake of fruits and vegetables.

- Find ways to stay active: Physical activity is an important part of maintaining a healthy weight and overall health. Aim to incorporate at least 150 minutes of moderate-intensity physical activity or 75 minutes of vigorous-intensity physical activity into your weekly routine, as recommended by the Centers for Disease Control and Prevention (CDC). This can include activities such as walking, running, cycling, swimming, or participating in group fitness classes.
- Manage stress: Chronic stress can contribute to weight gain and can make it more challenging to maintain a healthy weight. Find ways to manage stress, such as through relaxation techniques, exercise, or seeking support from friends and family.
- Build a supportive network: Having a supportive network of friends, family, and healthcare professionals can be incredibly helpful as you work towards your weight loss goals. A supportive network can provide encouragement, motivation, and guidance as you navigate the challenges of weight loss and maintenance.
- Stay consistent: Consistency is key when it comes to maintaining a healthy weight. Rather than trying to make dramatic changes all at once, focus on making small, sustainable changes that you can stick to over the long term. This can help to build healthy habits that can support long-term weight loss and overall health.
- Monitor your progress: Regularly monitoring your

progress can be helpful in maintaining your weight loss. This can involve keeping track of your weight, measuring your waist circumference, or keeping a food diary to track your intake. Regular monitoring can help you identify any potential challenges or areas for improvement, and can help you stay on track towards your goals.

- Don't be too hard on yourself: It's important to be kind and understanding towards yourself as you work towards your weight loss goals. Setbacks and challenges are a normal part of the process, and it's important to be patient and to focus on the progress you have made, rather than dwelling on any setbacks or failures. It can be helpful to practice self-compassion and to remind yourself that everyone makes mistakes, and that it's okay to ask for help when you need it.

By making sustainable lifestyle changes, staying active, managing stress, building a supportive network, and staying consistent, you can maintain your weight loss and build healthy habits for the long haul. Remember to be kind to yourself, and to focus on the progress you have made, and to seek out help when you need it. With the right mindset and approach, you can maintain your weight loss and enjoy improved overall health and well-being.

www.ingramcontent.com/pod-product-compliance
Lightning Source LLC
LaVergne TN
LVHW052115160826
845678LV00015B/3570

* 9 7 9 8 3 7 1 3 7 7 4 3 2 *